DIY Homemade Medical Face Mask

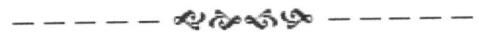

How to Make Your Own Virus Protection Mask in Less Than 15 Minutes for Less Than $1 a Piece!

By Matthew Anderson

Copyright © 2020 Matthew Anderson

All rights reserved.

All rights reserved. No part of this guide may be reproduced in any form without permission in writing from the publisher except in the case of brief quotations embodied in critical articles or reviews.

Legal & Disclaimer

The information contained in this book and its contents is not designed to replace or take the place of any form of medical or professional advice; and is not meant to replace the need for independent medical, financial, legal or other professional advice or services, as may be required. The content and information in this book has been provided for educational and entertainment purposes only.

The content and information contained in this book has been compiled from sources deemed reliable, and it is accurate to the best of the Author's knowledge, information and belief. However, the Author cannot guarantee its accuracy and validity and cannot be held liable for any errors and/or omissions. Further, changes are periodically made to this book as and when needed. Where appropriate and/or necessary, you must consult a professional (including but not limited to your doctor, attorney, financial advisor or such other professional advisor) before using any of the suggested remedies, techniques, or information in this book.

Upon using the contents and information contained in this book, you agree to hold harmless the Author from and against any damages, costs, and expenses, including any legal fees potentially resulting from the application of any of the information provided by this book. This disclaimer applies to any loss, damages or injury caused by the use and application, whether directly or indirectly, of any advice or information presented, whether for breach of contract, tort, negligence, personal injury, criminal intent, or under any other cause of action.

You agree to accept all risks of using the information presented inside this book.

You agree that by continuing to read this book, where appropriate and/or necessary, you shall consult a professional (including but not limited to your doctor, attorney, or financial advisor or such other advisor as needed) before using any of the suggested remedies, techniques, or information in this book.

Table of Contents

Introduction to DIY Homemade Medical Face Mask 6

    How to Wear a Mask Correctly 7

Chapter 1: Types of face masks 10

Chapter 2: How effective are face masks and respirators? 14

Chapter 3: How to make a surgical face mask at home? 17

    How does a mask work? 18

Chapter 4: How to wear different types of face masks? 19

Chapter 5: How to make a medical facemask .. 21

    Guidelines 25

Chapter 6: Other Ways of Protecting Yourself from Bacteria 31

Conclusion 34

Introduction to Making Your Own Hand Sanitizer 40

Chapter 1: Does Hand Sanitizers Work Against Viruses? 43

Composition of Hand Sanitizers 45

Chapter 2: Basic Ingredients Required to Make a Hand Sanitizer 46

Aromatherapy Add-ons............... 47

How Does sanitizer Work? 51

Chapter 3: Gathering the Necessary Equipment 52

Chapter 4: Various types of hand sanitizers 54

Chapter 5: Five ways to make a homemade sanitizer............... 62

Gentle Hand Sanitizer Formula (Safe for Kids) 62

Stronger Hand Sanitizer Formula............... 62

Strongest Homemade Hand Sanitizer Formula (5 Minute Formula)............... 64

Witch Hazel-Based Hand Sanitizer 65

The One Thing That Is THE ABSOLUTE BEST Germ Destroyer on The Planet (And Is As Cheap As A Bottle Of Water) 67

What to look on when you buy disinfectant 67

How to make your own disinfectant............... 68

Conclusion 70

Introduction to DIY Homemade Medical Face Mask

In this guide we will show you how to make 2 different types of protective face masks at home using easily available materials and with simple steps that anyone can do without special skills. In this period of virus pandemic emergency this practical guide could save the lives of many people since the masks on the market may not be enough for everyone and difficult to find in stores.

First of all is very important to know what are the various masks categories on the market, their protective characteristics and their differences. After that we will describe the necessary steps to make a mask at home which obviously is not certified like those on the market but which has almost the same characteristics. Reading this guide, we can all contribute to the protection from infection with appropriate precautions and anyone can wear his mask without worrying about not being able to buy one.

How to Choose the Right Face Mask? Differences and main categories The first thing you need to know is that the masks differ in 2 macro categories: those to protect against viruses and those to protect people from chemical and dangerous substances present in some works.

In this emergency situation both are used. Filtering masks against micro particles present in the air and toxic substances are very common in working environments and are divided into 3 protection classes: FFP1, FFP2 and FFP3 where the abbreviation FFP stands for "Filtering Face Piece". These masks are mandatory in environments where the limit value of the maximum contraction of dust, smoke and aerosol in the air is exceeded (OEL: Occupational Exposure Limit).

Surgical masks and other models such as the N95 are often used in medical and hospital environments. We see below the characteristics of these masks and the categories of use.

How to Wear a Mask Correctly

Correctly wearing a mask is an effective means to block the spread of respiratory secretions. The selection of medical surgical masks can prevent the spread of respiratory diseases. Wear it as follows: Wash your hands before wearing a mask, and avoid touching the inside of the mask with your hand during wearing the mask to reduce the possibility of the mask being polluted;

when wearing, clearing distinguish the inside and outside of the mask, the top and bottom, the light-colored surface is inside, the dark-colored side is facing outward, and one end of the metal strip(nose clip) is above the mask, fully unfold the folded surface;

put the side with the nose clip up, shield the outh, nose, lower jaw and adjust the down end of the mask to the proper position of the lower jaw, hang the elastic bands on both sides of the ears, or tie the two end bands behind the head, and then squeeze the nose clip so that the mask fits without a glitch on the face.

How to Wear N95 Mask

Wearing method: "N95" mask (head-mounted)

Hold the mask with one hand, the side with the metal sheet facing up

First, pull the lower strap over the head and place it under the ears behind the neck

Pull the upper strap back over the neck and ears

Compact the metal nose clip to the shape of the bridge of the nose so that the mask fits the face

Airtightness test:

Cover the protective mask with both hands completely and exhale quickly. If there is dew near the nose clip, adjust the nose clip. If the air leak is around, adjust it so as not to leak.

How to Wear the Medical Mask

Wearing method of mask: (ear-hook type)

The colored face of the mask faces outwards, and the side with the metal sheet faces upwards. Try not to touch the outside with your hands before touching the inside to avoid cross-contamination of bacteria.

Chapter 1: Types of face masks

Surgical Masks: These are the most common masks that you see around, in the news, on the faces of people are mostly surgical face masks. Doctors, dentists and nurses often use this while treating their patients, mainly because these protect them from getting germs. Surgical masks can protect others from a patient suffering from any infectious disease. If any patient is wearing a surgical mask, and he coughs or sneezes, the mask doesn't allow the droplets to escape in the air around. But on the other hand, it doesn't protect you from getting infection if you are healthy. That's why health experts suggest that a surgical face mask should be worn by patients, not healthy people.

These masks are relatively thin and loose-fitted. The tiny droplets that come out with cough and sneeze (known as bioaerosols) containing the disease causing microbes are even tinier than the pores of this surgical mask and these droplets can seep through the parts of the mask. So, whereas they are helpful in stopping pathogens to escape if a patient wears them, they can't fully protect you if you are healthy and you face a patient with infectious disease who is not wearing it. In this way, surgical face masks are not a way of protection for healthy people.

In a nutshell, these masks are advisable to wear by the sick people to prevent spreading the disease.

Surgical face masks are disposable and are advised to use one time only.

N95 Respirators: Doctors and nurses who treat patients infected with any infectious disease use respirators. These are the same respirators which the construction workers use to protect themselves at work site. These respirators are heavy duty and designed to cover the face fully. They are air tight and can help you protect from getting infected to at least 95%. They can fit over your nose and mouth. CDC claims that these respirators, if worn properly, can filter out about 95% of particles and microorganisms those can use air as medium to travel. However, these respirators are not able to filter vapours, toxic gases and smoke. Yet, they are not full secure as they may allow 5% of particles to pass through which may cause infection. But 5% is a rare chance and though they can't promise a hundred percent protection, but a little precaution is much better than having no protection at all.

N95 masks can easily filter particles which are less than 0.3 micrometers. They are designed to filter particles like fumes, dust, aerosols, mists and smoke. They also can protect you against biological particles like pollen, animal dander, allergens, mold spores, and microorganisms. You can trust these respirators for protection against aerosol particles like cough or sneeze droplets that you can't see with your naked eyes.

Though they have a few limitations, for example, they do not fit on the little faces of children. If you have beards, long mustachios, or stubble, these respirators will not fit properly and protection will be compromised.

It is always advisable to practice wearing these respirators beforehand because a first time user may face difficulties in wearing them. A prior practice will prepare you to use them properly in the time of emergency.

P100 Respirator: These are also known as gas mask. You can reuse them. These masks are designed to protect people involved in woodworking, those who face exposure to lead, solvents, asbestos and chemicals. They are considered the safest mode of protection, filtering out all oil and non-oil particles to 97.99%.

Full Face Respirators: These respirators cover your full face. These can protect you from gases and vapours. These not only protects you from inhaling the particles of gases or vapour but also protect them entering your eyes. You can reuse them. Though these respirators are much safer than all N, P, R respirators, these are very costly and therefore, it is not in the range of common people.

Self-contained breathing apparatuses: Basically, these are the most advanced type of face masks. They not only cover your whole face, but also have a breathing apparatuses with them. These help firefighters while they are on a mission to put out fire. These mask save them from dangerously polluted air.

Chapter 2: How effective are face masks and respirators?

Out of all the five categories given above, the respirators like N95, P100 have other variations, like N99, N100. The letter N is replaced by R and P in other variations. These letters and numbers tell us how effective a respirator is. Here you should understand that respirators are safer than a surgical mask because they are not air-tight, but the respirators are, and hence these are more protective in situations, than the surgical face masks.

The letters N, R, and P tells us if the mask can stop oil particles or not. N respirators are not resistant to oil based particles while, R respirators are resistant. N respirators are most common; they can be used for longer time and can protect you from smoke, particles in air, while R respirators have a short service life. R respirators are needed to change after eight hours because of clogging.

The P respirators are more effective than the others. They are classified as oil proof. But then, they are also not reusable, though they have longer use time. You may need to replace them after a total of 40 hours of use. They can be used in more dangerous situations.

The numbers 95, 99 and 100 tells us their efficiency in filtering particles. 95 rated respirators are effective in filtering 95% of particles, while 99 rated respirators can filter 99% of particles. The 100 rates respirators are not hundred percent efficient. They can filter only 99.97% particles.

If we look into protection, you can easily guess that P100 is the most effective mask that can filter both, non-oil and oil particles to 99.97%.

However, as all these respirators don't provide a 100% protection, you can understand that a 0.03% of exposure to deadly particles can harm you. But chances are rare. A little protection is better than nothing at all. Why taking any chance by not using face masks or respirators.

Here we should understand that all masks are not effective against all types of pathogens. World Health Organization and CDC recommends that two types of masks are effective in protecting you from lethal pathogens. These are surgical face mask and N95 respirator. Surgical face masks and N95 respirators are easily available around at chemist shops and also you can create them at your home if you don't find any in the market. However it is not advisable to try making an N95 respirator at home because you may not create them in the way to fully seal your face and chances of infection are higher. You should only buy these respirators created by trusted medical equipments creators.

Also, the other type of face masks like a full face respirator, have a high costs. It will not be possible for everyone to buy them.

World Health Organization and CDC recommend surgical face masks and N95 respirators for common people and health workers to avoid getting infected from pathogens. Whereas a N95 mask can have technicalities that it would be difficult and also not recommended to prepare at home, surgical masks are simple and you can create them at home in dire time of emergency. So, let's know how we can create a surgical face mask at home.

Chapter 3: How to make a surgical face mask at home?

During any dire emergency or during your normal life, you can wear a face mask as an extra protection even if you are healthy. For this, you can create a face mask for your own and can also contribute to the shortage.

CDC says that you can create homemade masks in the times of emergency but only as a last resort. These masks should be in combination with a face shield that should cover your entire frontal face, including chin and below and the sides of the face.

A study shows that cotton t-shirts and cotton pillowcases can be used to make effective face masks. You can easily breathe in these types of cloths and they can capture particles better than other types of cloths. They are as effective as surgical face masks.

Keep in mind, the edges of a mask should fit closely around your face, so that no respiratory droplets should invade.

To create a face mask, you can use piece of cotton t-shirts and pillowcases. They are easier to breathe. Use double layer of them. It will be protective and breathable. Fold them around the size of your mouth, and sew making folds in the cloth, just like stairs. Add elastic bands in the corners in U shape so that it can be worn in both ears.

You can add extra cloth to cover your chin also.

Though it should be understood that these homemade masks may not be able to provide a complete protection but a little effort can turn into success and a life can be saved. There is something always better than nothing.

How does a mask work?

The microbes and dust particles can be stopped to some extent by face masks. Let's know how does a face mask stops these so that you can understand properly, while creating a face mask.

Mostly the respirators filter the particles on the basis of many scientific principles, like gravitational settling, interception, diffusion, inertial impaction, and electrostatic deposition.

Filtering efficiency depends on the size of particles, charge concentration and rate of flow through the filtering material. However, the particles may bypass the filter by entering through the small gaps between the edge of masks and your face, known as the edge-seal leakage.

Chapter 4: How to wear different types of face masks?

It is recommended that before wearing a face mask you should wash your hands properly with soap and water or using an alcohol based hand sanitizer. CDC and WHO recommends using a hand sanitizer having at least 60% of alcohol to kill the pathogens.

After you wash your hands, take the mask from the box and you should check it if there are any tears or holes in any side of it.

To wear it, you should see which side of the mask is the front. Usually, the coloured side is the front of the mask and should face away from you. The white side should be towards you.

Follow these instructions to wear it properly:

Face mask with ear loops: To wear surgical face masks those come with ear loops, you should simply place the loops around your ears.

Face mask with ties: To wear such masks you should bring the mask to your nose and then place the ties over the crown of your head and secure it with a bow.

Face mask with bands: To wear masks with bands, simply bring it close to your nose and pull the top strap over your head in such a way that it should rest over the crown of your head. Now, pull the bottom strap over your head so that it can rest at the nape of your neck.

You should pinch or mold the edge to the shape of your nose.

If you are using a face mask with ties, you should secure it with a bow at the nape of your neck. You should pull the bottom of the mask over your mouth and chin.

The mask should closely fit your face. If you will be careless about covering your face you can get the infection. The mask lining should be sticking to your cheeks but it should not be tight on your nose or mouth. If the mask is tight on your nose, you will take the air more forcefully and in this effort, the pathogens will suck up inside the mask.

You should not touch the mask with your hands without washing them as your hands can have pathogens that can be transferred to the mask and later can be sucked up by your nose or mouth.

Chapter 5: How to make a medical facemask

Materials needed

The materials needed for large and medium size masks include two yards of 44-inch wide fabric, and four 18-inch ties. That much fabric should be able to make about 18 medium size masks or 15 big size masks.

For the outer layer of the mask, heavily tightly-woven 100 percent cotton is suggested but any tightly-woven durable 100 percent cotton fabric will still work.

In the inner layer, any tightly-woven 100 percent cotton fabric will do.

All fabrics must be 100 percent cotton that is pre-washed and pre-shrunk.

All seams should be sewn with a 3/8-inch allowance, which is typically the outside edge of the sewing machine foot. The top stitching should be close to the outer edge of the mask to help hold its shape.

The two pieces of the lining should be sewn together on the large curved side of the pieces with the right sides of the fabric inside.

Before sewing the outer and inner layers together, fold the fabric over 1/4 of an inch, then fold over 1/4 of an inch again, and top stitch near the edge of the fold.

Then, pin the inner and outer layers together.

Once that's done, the mask should be turned inside out. Then fold the edges of the outer layer even with the top and bottom edges of the mask. The sides should be folded 1/4 of an inch twice.

Put the unfinished end of the tie about 1/2 inch into the fold and top stitch the length of the side of the mask.

Once the ties are sewn, press all the edges of the face mask. Once that is done, top stitch the top and bottom edges of the mask close to the outer edges.

Then the mask is done.

How to sew a patterned surgical hospital mask

Many manufacturers have asked for a pattern for sewing homemade surgical masks for hospitals. The diy pattern in this book would show you how to make a standard pleated mask with elastic earmuffs.

This pattern consists of 2 layers of fabric and an inside pocket, in which you can add additional layers of disposable filter material if desired.

An important distinction

Homemade masks are not as effective as the cd95-recommended n95 filter mask and are not a substitute for proper ppe.

What fabric can you use to make a mask?

The best options for diy fabric masks are cotton t-shirts, pillow cases, or other cotton materials. I would be using a very high quality quilted cotton fabric for this pattern.

Using a double layer of material for your diy mask slightly increases filtration efficiency

Diy surgical mask pattern

Materials

- 100% cotton (with a tight weave)
- 1/8 "flat elastic or additional connective tissue
- Fabric scissors
- Ruler
- Pens or clips
- Sewing machine and thread

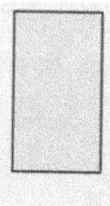 Cut one cotton rectangle, 8.5" wide by 15.5" long. Cut 2 7" pieces of elastic or 4 18" fabric strips.

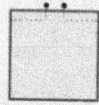 Fold in half and sew along the top, leaving a 2" opening for the pocket.

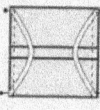 Sandwich the elastic or ties between the layers of fabric at the corners, and sew along each side to secure.

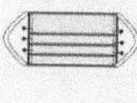 Turn the mask right side out. Fold 3 evenly-spaced 1/2" pleats. Pin in place, and sew to secure.

Cut list

For an adult size mask:

Cut 1 rectangle of fabric 15.5 "long and 8.5" wide

Cut 2 pieces of elastic, each 7 "long

For a child mask:

Cut 1 rectangle of fabric 13.5 "long by 6.5" wide

Cut 2 pieces of elastic, each 6 "long

For elastic earmuffs:

Cut 2 pieces 7 "long for an adult mask

Next step is for you to cut 2 pieces 6 "long for a child mask

For cloth ties if you are not wearing a rubber band:

Cut 4 rectangles 18 "long and 1.75" wide. Fold the long sides so that they meet in the middle, and then fold them in half again to enclose the raw edges. Sew along the rectangles along the edge to create the bindings.

Guidelines

Step 1: sew up with the pocket

Fold the fabric in half, with the right s are facing each other.

Sew along the 8.5 "wide edge with a 3/8" seam allowance. Leave a 2-3 inch opening in the middle of this seam to create an opening for the filter bag and let the mask turn outwards after sewing.

Don't you want a filter bag? If you don't want or need a bag, that's perfectly fine. Simply sew the seam completely and leave no opening free. Then you can continue with the remaining instructions.

Step 2: elastic pin

Twist the fabric so that the seam is with the bag

The opening is centered in the middle of one side. (if you haven't made a pocket opening, just skip this step and continue with the rubber band.)

Optionally, you can sew to reinforce the seam: press the open seam and the top stitch or the zigzag stitch along both sides of the seam to get a cleaner edge. Hold the mask upside down.

Put a piece of rubber band on the top and bottom of the short side of the fabric rectangle to create an earring. Place the ends of the rubber band 1/2 "from the top and bottom of the fabric.

The length of the rubber band is in the two layers of fabric so that it is on the outside when the mask is removed.

Repeat this process on the opposite side.

Option b: use fabric binders:

If you can't find elastic bands or prefer to use cloth ties, you can use 4 cloth ties, one on each corner. Each tie will be 18 "long. Sew a tie at each corner, being careful not to get the ties caught in the side seams.

The finished mask is worn by tying the strips of fabric behind the head.

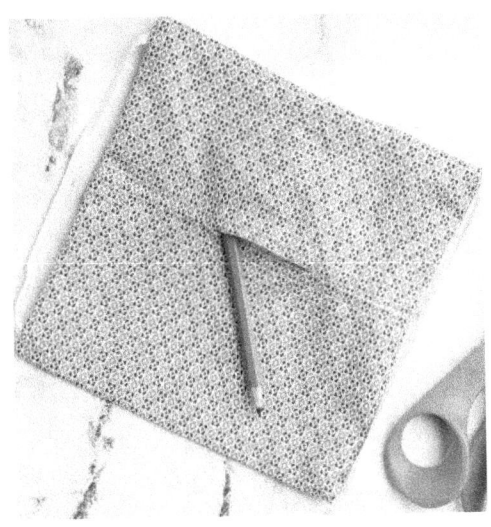

Step 3: sew the sides

Sew the sides of the mask. Sew over rubber bands or fabric bands to secure them. Cut the corners with scissors.

Fold out the mask and press with an iron. You can pull out the corners with a pencil.

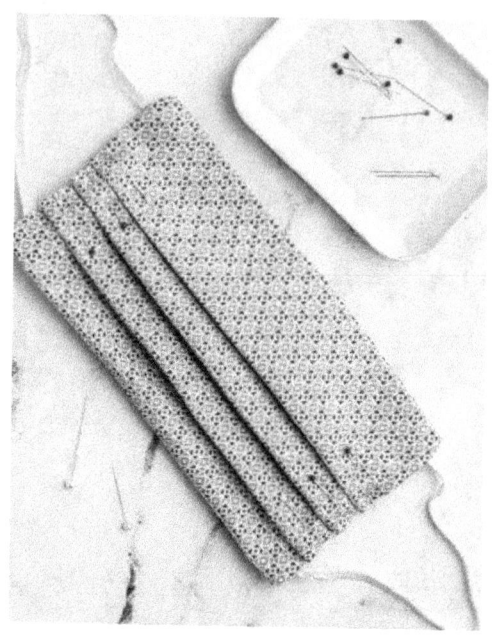

Step 4: make the folds

Create three 1/2-inch folds evenly spaced. Pin the folds and sew them along the sides. Make sure all folds are facing the same direction.

The finished mask will be approximately 3.75 inches tall.

When using the mask, the folds should open down to prevent particles from accumulating in the folding pockets.

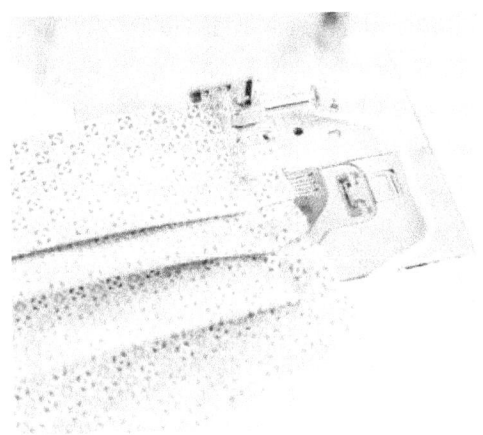

Troubleshoot the pattern

Can't find elastic?

I have heard from many people who have difficulty finding rubber bands. If you can't find the rubber band for the earmuffs, you can make a mask out of fabric bands. You can use a finished 1/4 "twill tape or double-fold tape, or cut long strips of the same tight cotton that you use for the rest of the mask.

How to make cloth bows: cut strips of cloth 18 "long, 1.75" wide. Fold the long sides together (lengthways or hot dog style) so that they meet in the middle. Then fold the strips in half again (lengthways) to enclose the raw edges. Sew the straps along the edge to make the ties.

If you want these straps to be a little stretchy, you can also cut long strips of cotton jersey or knit jersey material.

Whichever option you choose, you want to cut 4 pieces approximately 18 inches long and attach a strap to each corner. The mask is attached by tying the straps behind the head.

What about metal to make it fit better?

To make the mask fit better around your nose, you can insert a flexible metal length into the mask through the pocket insert opening at the top before forming the folds. You can then sew around the metal insert to hold it in place. I have seen people using pipe cleaners, flower wires or cable ties.

Chapter 6: Other Ways of Protecting Yourself from Bacteria

When it comes to protecting yourself from bacteria, there is never enough methods that will keep you safe. Wearing a face mask is just never enough. Bacteria is detrimental to health and can spread quickly. Good hand hygiene practice is necessary at this point. Since microbes and germs stays in the hand, it is essential that you keep it clean at all times. Washing hands with soap and water or with a hand sanitizer, together with putting on a medical face mask is an effective combination in combating bacteria.

Not all bacteria are harmful. Some bacteria in the intestine like Lactobacillus acidophilus helps in the digestion of food and destroys disease-causing organisms. Washing your hands is simple. However, if you don't wash it the correct way, there is a possibility that some germs are still lingering in one part of your hand. Follow these simple steps to wash your hands effectively with soap and water.

- Wet your hands with clean running water. Turn the tap off and apply soap.

- Rub your hands together with the soap until it forms lather. Lather the backs of your hands, in-between the fingers, and under the nails. Make sure you lather all parts of your hands.

- Scrub your hands like that between 15 - 20 seconds.

- Once you are done scrubbing, rinse your hands well under the running water.

Dry your hands with a clean towel.

In the absence of soap and water, you can use alcohol-based hand sanitizer. Alcohol-based sanitizers are not 100% effective against certain germs and harmful chemicals like pesticides. However, they are good alternatives to handwashing. In case you don't know how to wash your hands with a sanitizer, follow these simple steps.

- Ensure your hands are visibly dry.

- Apply the recommended amount in one palm and rub it together with the other. • Rub in-between the fingers and make sure your entire hands are well covered.

Once skin is dry, stop rubbing the sanitizer. Always put hand sanitizer in your bag because soap and water are not always available. This will keep you prepared for any eventuality. While you may think that washing hands and wearing a face mask are two vital ways of protecting yourself from bacteria, there are other couple of ways you can also protect yourself from germs. Other ways of protecting yourself from bacteria include:

Clean All Kitchen Utensils and Equipment - Kitchen hygiene is crucial in protecting you from bacteria. Eating unsafe food is one of the fastest way of contracting bacteria. So, you need to make sure that you prepare your food safely. Wash raw meat, fish, with salt. Clean utensils, tools, and kitchen counters.

• Practice Good Hygiene - Ensuring that you have all-round hygiene is critical. Make sure you wash your clothes and bed sheets all the time. Bacteria can hide in them for days and when you wear them without washing, you get infected. Bathe and brush your tooth for at least twice a day. Keep your environment clean. Clean all surfaces in the home, trim all tall grasses if you have any and empty the bins regularly. Bacterial can infest in all these and get transferred by the air to you.

• Drink Enough Water - Research has shown that drinking water after you are up in the morning will kickstart your body functions and prepare it for the day. Drinking enough water also helps to keep your skin smooth and prevent dryness. Drinking 2 - 3 liters of water per day will help boost the immune system and fight against bacteria.

Conclusion

When wearing a medical mask, you should select the suitable level according to the type of transmission of the pollutant and the risk. Although the medical protective mask with high protection level has a better protection effect, due to the high filter material level, good adhesion, and higher breathing resistance, long-term wearing will amplify the problem of breathing and other discomforts.

Medical-surgical masks and medical protective masks can wedge the toxins emitted by blood and body fluid splashes, on the other hand if you need to block the contamination of airborne particles and pathogenic microorganisms, choose to wear medical protective masks.

Medical-surgical masks can block most bacteria and some viruses, prevent medical staff from being infected and prevent medical staff from transmitting pathogenic bacteria to the outside world. Therefore, it is suitable for the basic protection of clinical medical staff; that is, it is used for clinical medical staff during invasive operation. Wear it in the middle to protect the treated patients and medical personnel performing invasive operations to prevent the spread of blood, body fluids, and splashes.
During the epidemic of infectious diseases, in relatively densely populated places, such as hospital

clinics or consultation offices, elevators, emergency departments, etc., medical-surgical masks can effectively prevent the spread of pathogenic bacteria and play a preventive and protective role for various types of personnel.

Making Your Own Hand Sanitizer

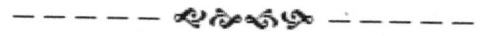

Protect Yourself Against The Virus – How To Make 500 Ml. Of Hand Sanitizer In Just 25 Minutes!

By Health's First Products & Samantha Johnson

Copyright © 2020 Health's First Products & Samantha Johnson

All rights reserved.

All rights reserved. No part of this guide may be reproduced in any form without permission in writing from the publisher except in the case of brief quotations embodied in critical articles or reviews.

Legal & Disclaimer

The information contained in this book and its contents is not designed to replace or take the place of any form of medical or professional advice; and is not meant to replace the need for independent medical, financial, legal or other professional advice or services, as may be required. The content and information in this book has been provided for educational and entertainment purposes only.

The content and information contained in this book has been compiled from sources deemed reliable, and it is accurate to the best of the Author's knowledge, information and belief. However, the Author cannot guarantee its accuracy and validity and cannot be held liable for any errors and/or omissions. Further, changes are periodically made to this book as and when needed. Where appropriate and/or necessary, you must consult a professional (including but not limited to your doctor, attorney, financial advisor or such other professional advisor) before using any of the suggested remedies, techniques, or information in this book.

Upon using the contents and information contained in this book, you agree to hold harmless the Author from and against any damages, costs, and expenses, including any legal fees potentially resulting from the application of any of the information provided by this book. This disclaimer applies to any loss, damages or injury caused by the use and application, whether directly or indirectly, of any advice or information presented, whether for breach of contract, tort, negligence, personal injury, criminal intent, or under any other cause of action.

You agree to accept all risks of using the information presented inside this book.

You agree that by continuing to read this book, where appropriate and/or necessary, you shall consult a professional (including but not limited to your doctor, attorney, or financial advisor or such other advisor as needed) before using any of the suggested remedies, techniques, or information in this book.

Introduction to Making Your Own Hand Sanitizer

Hands, if or not ungloved, are among the chief methods of spreading disease or for moving bacterial contamination. The usage of hand disinfectants is a part of the procedure for fantastic pollution control for employees working in hospital surroundings, or people involved with aseptic processing and inside cleanrooms. Even though there are lots of distinct sorts of hand sanitizers accessible that there are differences using their efficacy, and many don't match the European standard available sanitization.

Employees operating in hospitals and cleanrooms take various kinds of microorganisms in their palms, and these germs can be easily transferred from person to person or by individual to gear or surfaces that are critical. For critical surgeries, some security is given by sporting gloves. However, gloves aren't appropriate for many gloves and activities or even frequently sanitized or, if they're of an improper layout, can pick up and move contamination.

Hence, the sanitization of palms (either gloved or ungloved) is an equally significant part contamination management in hospitals, to steer clear of staff-to-patient cross-contamination or before undertaking surgical or clinical procedures; and also, for aseptic trainings such as the dispensing of medications. Additionally, not only is that the usage of a hand sanitizer required before undertaking these programs, it's likewise essential that the sanitizer is good at removing a large population of germs. Various studies have revealed that when a very low number of germs persist following the use of a sanitizer; subsequently, the subpopulation can grow, which can be resistant to potential programs.

There are lots of commercially available hand sanitizers having the most frequently used forms being alcohol-based fluids or dyes. Much like other varieties of disinfectants, hand sanitizers are effective against different germs based upon their style of action. Together with the most typical alcohol-based hand sanitizers, the manner of activity contributes to bacterial cell passing through cytoplasm leakage, denaturation of protein, and ultimate cell lysis (alcohols are among those so-called 'membrane disrupters'). The benefits of using alcohols as hand sanitizers incorporate a comparatively low price, small odor, and a fast evaporation (restricted residual activity contributes to shorter contact times). Additionally, alcohols have an established cleansing activity.

In picking a hands sanitizer, the pharmaceutical business or clinic will have to think about whether the program will be forced into human skin to gloved hands or to either, and if it's necessary to become sporicidal. Hand sanitizers fall into two different classes: alcohol established, which can be more prevalent, and also non-alcohol based. Such factors affect both upon price as well as the health and security of the employees utilizing the hand sanitizer because most generally accessible alcohol-based sanitizers may lead to excessive drying of the skin; and also a few non-alcohols established sanitizers may be irritating to skin. Alcohol hand sanitizers are intended to prevent irritation through owning sterile properties (color and odor-free) and components that manage skin protection and attention via re-fatting agents.

Alcohols have a lengthy history of usage as disinfectants as a result of inherent antiseptic properties from bacteria and some viruses. To succeed, some water must be blended with alcohol to apply effect against germs, together with the very best variety falling between 60 and 95 percent (most industrial hand sanitizers are approximately 70 percent). The most widely used alcohol-based hand sanitizers have been Isopropyl alcohol or some type of denatured ethanol (for instance, Industrial Methylated Spirits). The more prevalent non-alcohol established sanitizers include either chlorhexidine or hexachlorophene. Additives may also be contained in hand sanitizers so as to grow the anti-inflammatory properties.

Chapter 1: Does Hand Sanitizers Work Against Viruses?

Before offering recipes for making natural antibacterial gel, we want to clarify what its properties are. This type of gels has antibacterial properties, so they kill a variety of bacteria they also have fungicidal properties, that is, they eliminate pathogenic fungi, and they are also powerful disinfectants, eliminating a wide variety of germs. But what about viruses?

As indicated by the WHO, antibacterial gels are not suitable against viruses, as they are bactericidal and not virucidal; just like with antibiotic drugs, they fight against bacteria, not against viruses. However, there are some disinfecting gels with a virucidal effect, and in this case, it is indicated on the product label.

Wash your hands thoroughly as indicated, you should start by using soap and water and then apply the gel to both hands thoroughly (both palms and backs and between fingers) and let it dry. The part of hand washing should last between 40 and 60 seconds and that of hand disinfection between 20 and 30 seconds. You should never use only gel; except you've washed with soap and water for a very short time or in places and situations where there is not good access to soap and water).

Using hand sanitizers by those that have a great deal of touch with the general public, together with regular hand washing machine, would really prevent illness. The practice is straightforward. Hand sanitizers include alcohol at a concentrated form. Alcohol kills germs. Microorganisms cause illness.

Among our major concerns within our wellbeing and retaining us emptiness of germs and fungal disease would be with the support of hand sanitizer dispensers. Considering all the mortal diseases and pandemics that we've struck previously, it's quite vital for all of us to remain secure and take care of the cleanliness of ourselves and our environment, not only on which our eyes can observe, but those who we can't.

In our everyday lives, we ought to know about where the contamination and spread of virus will be possible. Crowded and often seen places such as metro stations and other people are all sources of these germs which you might even choose home. It's then important to get a convenient hand sanitizer dispenser on your luggage when traveling. In case you've got enough opportunity to clean your hands if you visit a comfortable space, do this. This will also assist in protecting yourself from germs which you may get. When a hand sanitizer is offered at precisely the exact same rest space, avail yourself of this privilege.

Often handed down, things like coins and invoices are passed around can attract viruses. This cart that you have been pushing around the supermarket, the doorway from the diner, or the countertop at the lender could all have been managed with many people who you can not tell, which got you contaminated. It's then important to guard yourself in them being moved to you by massaging your hands after each managing.

Composition of Hand Sanitizers

In order to prepare hand sanitizers at home, it is important to know the basic ingredients that are required to make it effective against the germs. Hand sanitizers are 90 percent alcohol, and about ten percent of the other ingredients that are used to add color, scent, and texture. Hand sanitizers vary in forms, some are prepared as clear gel-like liquids, and some are foamy in appearance.

Chapter 2: Basic Ingredients Required to Make a Hand Sanitizer

Irrespective of the recipe used, the following are the basic ingredients and things that you will need to make a good hand sanitizer.

These ingredients are commonly available at the medical stores or you can also find them in the super stores under the label of different companies. It is important consider the percentages of the alcohol used.

99.9% isopropyl alcohol: Rubbing alcohol and simple alcohol is used to make the base of the sanitizer. Keep the rubbing alcohol stored in a sealed and tight container, then use only when all other ingredients of the hand sanitizer are ready to combine.

98% aloe Vera gel: To get a gel-like consistency, nothing works better than aloe Vera gel. You can either use fresh gel, directly extracted from the Aloe Vera leaves or the gel that is available in the market. Aloe Vera naturally has healing properties, and it is also great for the skin.

10 % Witch hazel: Liquid extracted from witch hazel plants and is used for its disinfectant properties. The liquid contains tannins that repair skin, heal wounds, and fight bacteria.

Drops of essential oils: Essential oils are basically added to give a particular fragrance to the sanitizer. You can use any one of the following essential oils and add only a few drops to each bottle of sanitizer:

Aromatherapy Add-ons

With all of the options that you have been given above, you should feel well-prepared to make your own hand sanitizer if need be. Whether the stores are all sold out or you simply want to switch to a homemade option, all of these recipes are simple to create. There are countless essential oil options for you to use to put a creative twist on any sanitizer that is plain or relatively unscented. The following guide can assist you when you are selecting your additional ingredients.

Cinnamon

Not only is it a delicious scent that most people enjoy, but cinnamon is also known to be effective at reducing drowsiness. This invigorating scent can be added to your hand sanitizer blends for an additional boost. It is also known for helping you stay focused, a great addition for hand sanitizer that you plan on bringing with you to work. If you are prone to headaches, the scent has also been known to relieve them. It is one of the most healing essential oils out there, for good reason.

Lavender

This scent has the opposite effects of cinnamon. Lavender oil is best known for its relaxing and calming properties. People enjoy this scent when they are trying to relax or stay calm. If you plan on keeping hand sanitizer on your bedside table, making a blend with lavender essential oil would be a great decision. This is also a great scent to use if you are making hand sanitizer for your children. Because it is not so harsh, kids also generally enjoy the smell while receiving the same calming effects.

Lemon

Lemon oil is another aromatherapy option that will leave you feeling rejuvenated and energized. It is a scent that most people enjoy in the morning because it is very fresh. Many individuals will make lemon-scented hand sanitizer that is kept in the kitchen. If you are feeling down or stressed, lemon oil can help you by easing these symptoms. Overall, it is a very beneficial scent that is also very familiar to most people. Because it is so potent, you won't need to use a lot of oil to achieve all of the benefits that it has to offer.

Peppermint

Best known for calming your nerves, peppermint is a relaxing scent that most people associate with the holidays. Because of its benefits, you can use it year-round. When you add peppermint oil to your hand sanitizer, you can anticipate a renewed feeling of mental clarity. It can allow you to concentrate better and stay focused on the things that are most important at the moment. This is a great addition to any sanitizer that you play on keeping with you in your bag because it can help you stay alert while you are driving. You will learn to appreciate the calmness, yet focus, that it provides.

Tea Tree

This is a very potent oil and some people do not enjoy how strong it smells. Tea tree oil is full of benefits, though. It is one of the most highly antiseptic and antibacterial essential oils which is why it makes a lot of sense to add it to your homemade hand sanitizer recipes. As it helps you to heal from inflammation, tea tree oil can also calm you down in the same way that peppermint can. If you are able to handle the smell, this can create a very effective hand sanitizer that you will feel confident in. You will notice an overall improvement in your mood and alertness.

Rosemary

Not as commonly used, rosemary oil is great with helping your memory. When you need to retain information, smelling something that contains rosemary oil before and after can help you. It gives you a pleasant scent, but because it is not as fruity or floral as other essential oils, it is less commonly selected for hand sanitizers. Mixing a little bit of rosemary oil with lemon oil can provide you with a rejuvenating blend if you do not want to use it on its own. The rosemary oil will ensure that you are alert and ready to retain any information that comes your way.

Geranium

A floral scent that is known for being relatively mild, adding geranium oil to your sanitizer can provide you with a pleasant smell without being too overpowering. Many people who are sensitive to strong scents enjoy using geranium oil because it is subtle. It is the most floral scent of the above oils, but when used sparingly, it can give your sanitizer just enough added scent without giving you a headache. Smelling geranium on a regular basis can lift your mood, allowing you to feel happier. It may also help relieve PMS symptoms. You will feel instantly relaxed when you smell this essential oil in your homemade hand sanitizer.

Aromatherapy is very important to consider when you are crafting your own hand sanitizer recipes. The more that you familiarize yourself with the process, the better you will feel about experimenting. Making your own hand sanitizer can be a fun process that allows everyone in the family to have their own custom blend. As you can see, essential oils do a lot more for the sanitizer than adding a pleasant scent to it. These oils provide additional benefits to your hand sanitizers, and you can choose the ones more useful or appropriate for you and your family.

How Does sanitizer Work?

Sanitizer kills the microorganisms against which it is used. Disinfectant has a denaturing effect, i.e., it changes the protein structures of the microorganisms. Some disinfectants also damage the membrane of the virus or the nucleic acids of the germs. The self-made disinfectants especially aim to change the protein-containing structures due to the alcohol they contain.

Chapter 3: Gathering the Necessary Equipment

For all the recipes in this book, you'll need either a jar or small bowl for mixing your sanitizer, measuring cups and spoons, and of course a spoon (or better yet, a whisk) for stirring. (You can certainly make larger batches by doubling or otherwise scaling up the amounts of ingredients if you're really planning to stock up, in which case you'll need a larger bowl!) A funnel can also be useful for transferring your sanitizer to a storage container without spilling. Avoiding contamination is also an issue here – all the equipment you're going to use to make your hand sanitizer, including bowls, spoons, jars, should be thoroughly cleaned and sanitized before use. In terms of storage, most people say that old, empty pump or squirt bottles get the job done just fine. For maximum convenience, you're definitely going to want a container that can easily dispense a consistent amount of sanitizer onto your hands, because as we'll discuss later, the amount you use is actually important. Also, make sure that whatever storage option you choose is air-tight to avoid having your sanitizer evaporate or spilling. If you are recycling an old product container, though, be sure to clean it out well, including the lid, nozzle, etc. and make sure to sanitize it before filling it with your sanitizer. One easy way to do this is to spray some rubbing alcohol inside the container and let it sit until the alcohol has evaporated. Also, don't forget to label your container so that no-one accidentally ingests your sanitizer. Having a piece of knowledge on how to make disinfectant is excellent because you can make from natural ingredients blended with essential oils, you can quickly achieve a natural viral and antibacterial effects. This means you are a terror to germs via your own handmade disinfectant as a regular bottle of hand sanitizer is always around you.

Chapter 4: Various types of hand sanitizers

There are different types of hand sanitizers and I explained few of them which is also the common one that you can make easily from your homes and the recipes for it can be easily seen in our kitchens and farms.

One of them is the alcoholic hand sanitizer which can be made by using some alcoholic substances like, ethanol, isopropyl with other ingredients to form the sanitizer. I really prefer using isopropyl because of its qualities. It is flammable and dries the skin completely after usage. It kills germs and bacteria faster and it is also added because of its strength to fight bacteria. It is very active and effective when used to make sanitizer and a certain amount in percentage is needed to boast the strength of the sanitizer and make it work efficiently. Another type of hand sanitizer that I will discuss about again is the nonalcoholic one that involves using other ingredients like aloe vera to produce it. Aloe vera is a special leaf that is nutrient and helps in fighting diseases as well, it has other natures like nourishing the body, keeping it refreshed and smooth. It works perfectly in this type of sanitizer when mixed with other substances like glycerol and mix completely with distilled water at a certain measurement and calculations.

It stays longer on the skin unlike the alcoholic based hand sanitizer and leaves the skin with a lovely sweet smell whenever it is applied on it.

But the alcohol-based sanitizer is considered to be more effective and work faster. There are other things added to it to make it soluble and they include the glycerol that I mentioned earlier which is a simple compound that odorless and colorless in nature, very viscous liquid, nontoxic and have a very smart taste though it can be used for making food but research showed also that it may lead to some side effects like headache, vomiting and even nausea when taking into the body system. But it is really good for making of various hand sanitizer because of those qualities in it.

So, when doing the alcohol-based hand sanitizer, always have in mind that it is inflammable and can burn in blue flame when in contact with fire so it must be kept out of it. This is to help you to be cautious about it by keeping it out from it and put it away from the reach of your kids.

The spray bottle is really needed to which will serve as the final collector.it is a bottle that has a nob for spraying and its very good for the sanitizer liquid to be able to control the usage of it in an appropriate way. It is necessary to wash before using to avoid some germs and bacteria hiding in it and contaminating the solution when it is poured inside. So, for you to wash it, you will first use the distilled water to wash thoroughly and then rinse it later with the alcohol because of the bacteria and germs for alcohol has the strength of killing every germs and bacteria that might be hiding in it. This is to make sure that you are using a completely free from germs bottle so that your sanitized solution be made pure and free from any form of contaminations.

It is very portable and you can carry it whenever and where you go. There will not be any damage to the skin when you use this but the perfect work is the ability to eliminate the microorganisms. From the skin and make sure it is protected and preserved from diseases caused by germs or bacteria.

It makes the skin to look fresh.it is advisable to monitor it to avoid wrong usage by the kids or anybody who does not really know what it is so after the production, you are advised to make a label and stick on it for precautions .

We have another substance called the essential oil or tea tree oil which is also needed to make the sanitizer and this is gotten when you steam the leaves of Australia tea tree. This oil is very good antibacterial and it is used for treating so many bacteria and germ causing diseases like lice.it is very good for the hand sanitizer because of its medicinal nature.

Another material for making the sanitizer is the hydrogen peroxide which can be said to be a very good antiseptic and is used to cure some infectious diseases of the skin. This is dangerous to health when taken in or consumed by very effective to the skin for killing diseases. This material is needed in the hand sanitizer to make it work effectively.

When It's Safe to Use Hand Sanitizer—and When You Need to Find Soap and Water

Yeah, we remember, you were told about a bazillion times during the cold and flu season, to wash your hands daily. A brief refresher on why it's so, so important: Virus-containing droplets expelled through sneezes or coughs can be easily transmitted between people— even by merely shaking hands or grabbing a doorknob and then touching your nose or mouth.

So even in those cases, a wash with soap and water is your best option (after a flu shot, of course), a sink isn't always readily available; often you can't just pry yourself away from your office, whether you're in the midst of an outdoor workout. "You can't just be in the bathroom washing your hands all day," says Pritish K. Tosh, MD, a physician and researcher at the Mayo Clinic for infectious disease.

Join the sanitizer by hand. The alcohol-based gel plays the role of a knight in shining armor for those of us who can't help scrub-a-dub-dub around the clock from what we are doing. "It seems like an excellent idea to use them because of their simplicity and effectiveness," Dr. Tosh agrees.

And sometimes the hand sanitizer is a good idea — as long as you obey certain basic rules.

If soap and water are not available, disinfect your hands with a hand sanitizer Washing your hands with soap and water is always the first line of protection against a host of disease-inducing species, Dr. Tosh says. But when you can't get it to the sink, hand sanitizer will battle specific bugs too, like cold-causing viruses and flu.

Nonetheless, a report published in the journal Pediatrics this week poses concerns about conditions where a hand sanitizer can be more successful than washing up. The study showed that young children were less likely to get sick and skip daycare when they were using hand sanitizer than when they were washing their hands.

"Since the use of hand sanitizers is also convenient, people might be more likely to do it and use so more frequently than anyone would just stick to soap and water," Dr. Tosh hypothesizes. "And though the effectiveness [of hand sanitizer] may be smaller, there may be greater overall potential to avoid infection as it's easier to do more often." However, he says, experts aren't giving us the green light to fully skip the sink.

Should not use hand sanitizer when your hands are filthy. According to the Centers for Disease Control and Prevention (CDC), when your hands are coated in the muck, sanitizers actually will not function as well — say after you've been planting or tinkering with your bike gears.

For example, if you just apply sanitizer to the mix, the dirt and grease won't go anywhere, says TanayaBhowmick, MD, assistant professor of infectious disease medicine at the Robert Wood Johnson Medical School in New Jersey. "When you've got dirt on your hands and put alcohol on it, you're just making a slurry." She says you're going to rub the gunk around without ever washing it off.

And because hand sanitizer doesn't destroy every microbe, she underlines that there are those that you just need to wash off.

Ensure sure the sanitizer is at least 60% alcohol. The alcohol serves as what's considered a denaturing agent, explains Dr. Tosh, as opposed to soap, which serves as a detergent. Essentially, alcohol destroys or inactivates viruses— and, according to the CDC, it does so most efficiently in sanitizers that are between 60 and 95 percent alcohol.

Proper application, Dr. Bhowmick adds, is also essential. Apply hand sanitizer to one hand's palm, then "keep rubbing around all your hands until it's warm," she says. Pleasant reminder: You shouldn't have your hand sanitizer cleaned off, whether you're using a towel or your jeans ' legs (hey, we were there). "It defeats the intent, because whatever you wipe it off on, you may be picking up something else," says Dr. Bhowmick.

We like the vegan Instant Hand Sanitizer from Noodle & Boo ($10, dermstore.com), and the Advanced Hand Sanitizer from Purell with aloe ($13 for 4, amazon.com). It's a wise idea to look for an alcohol-based sanitizer with a moisturizing agent like aloe, Dr. Tosh says, because all that alcohol will dry up.

Avoid something branded as "antibacterial" If you're an obsessive user of hand sanitizer, you may have wondered if you're too full of it. Luckily, gels based on alcohol will continue to work just as well over time, so keep on rubbing on. "At least up to now, there's no evidence suggesting this isn't as successful [over time]," Dr. Bhowmick says — at least when it comes to killing viruses. Some research indicates that drug-resistant bacteria can develop an alcohol tolerance, though, she says.

That's a little worrying, considering the ever-growing danger of microbial resistance— when bacteria evolve to survive the antibiotics usually used to kill them. Dr. Tosh says that overuse of antibacterial and antimicrobial products will bolster those so-called superbugs, so stay away from the hand gels on their labels that advertise those properties.

Chapter 5: Five ways to make a homemade sanitizer

Gentle Hand Sanitizer Formula (Safe for Kids)

A non-drying, natural hand sanitizer gel feeds on aloe vera. It's so easy to be able to help the kids make it.

Prepare Time: 1 minute

Ingredients:

- 1/4 cup aloe vera gel
- 20 drops destroyer germ essential oil

Directions

Combine all ingredients and store in a reusable silicone container.

Stronger Hand Sanitizer Formula

Using as needed to eliminate germs naturally from Stronger Hand Sanitizer Recipe. Use this recycle for a more reliable hand sanitizer that works like commercial versions (without the triclosan). If you're operating in a hospital, this might be a perfect one for personal use. This recycle I wouldn't use on kids!

Ingredients:

- 1 TBSP rubbing alcohol
- 1/2 tsp vegetable glycerin (optional)
- 1/4 cup aloe vera gel
- 20 drops Germ Destroyer oil
- 1 TBSP distilled water or colloidal silver / ionic silver for extra antibacterial activity
- Other essential oils (just for scent)

Directions

To produce, blend aloe vera gel, optional glycerin, and rub alcohol in a small bowl.

Add essential oil of cinnamon and tea tree oil along with a drop or two of any other oils that you wish to add for fragrance. Sweet options include lemongrass, peach, lavender, and peppermint.

Mix well and add about one tablespoon of distilled water (or ionic/colloidal silver) to thin consistency if desired.

To pass hand sanitizer into a spray or pump-style bottles, using a small funnel or medicine dropper. This can also be packed for use on the go in small silicone tubes.

Using any other form of hand sanitizer as you can.

Strongest Homemade Hand Sanitizer Formula (5 Minute Formula)

To effectively kill viruses, the CDC recommends at least 60 percent alcohol in hand sanitizer. This formula follows the percentage and adds aloe vera for gentleness and essential oils for the fight against new viruses. This is the one that I'm using after working in places where the transmission of infections is more likely.

Ingredients:

- 2/3 cup alcohol rubbing (70 percent or higher)
- 2 Teaspoons aloe vera (if aloe vera can not be found, glycerin may be used as a substitute)
- 20 drops Germ Destroyer Essential Oil (You can also use Germ Fighter which is more robust, but I wouldn't recommend it for use on kids)

Directions

Mix all the ingredients and combine them in a spray bottle (these are the best size) or any small container. Use as you wish.

Keep in mind that the formula should be changed according to the strength of the alcohol you're using. For example, if you're using 99% Isopropyl rubbing alcohol, you're going to need a different amount of aloe vera than if you're using 70% alcohol. Below are some fast guidelines.

Option 1 - with 99% Isopropyl Rubbing Alcohol: two parts of alcohol and one part of aloe vera gel (e.g., 2/3 cup alcohol + 1/3 cup aloe vera gel).

Option 2 - with 91% isopropyl or rubbing alcohol: three parts whiskey and one part aloe vera gel (e.g., 3/4 cup alcohol + 1/4 cup aloe vera gel).

Option 3 - with 70% isopropyl or rubbing alcohol: nine parts of alcohol and one part of aloe vera gel.

Some people tend not to use alcohol in their hand sanitizer because alcohol has a strong odor and can have a significant drying effect on the skin.

Witch Hazel-Based Hand Sanitizer

A perfect option is the use of a witch-hazel-based sanitizer. The tea tree oil has additional antiseptic benefits.

Ingredients:

- 1 cup (preferably without additives) of pure aloe vera gel
- 1/2 teaspoons hazel 30 drops tea tree oil five drops of essential oil like lavender or peppermint Spoon Funnel Glass bottle

Directions

Stir in aloe vera water, tea tree oil, and hazel witch. To thicken it, add another spoonful of aloe vera if the mixture is too thin. Remove another spoonful of witch hazel.

If it is too thick, stir the essential oil in. Since the tea tree oil's scent is already stable, the added essential oils are simple to handle. Five or so drops are meant to be enough, but mix it in one drop at a time if you want to add more.

Funn the mixture into the receptacle. Place the funnel above the jar mouth and pour in the sanitizer for the side. Fill it up, then screw it onto the lid until ready to use it.

A tiny bottle of squirt works well if you want to take the sanitizer with you all day long.

Save the remaining sanitizer in a container with a tightly fitting lid, if you make too much for the bottle.

The One Thing That Is THE ABSOLUTE BEST Germ Destroyer on The Planet (And Is As Cheap As A Bottle Of Water)

Ok. Straightforward – that is CHLORINE. And it is very good for disinfecting the commonly used surfaces like office table, dining table, and whatever you constantly touch in your hose.

Chlorine is recommended by the World Organization of Health. It is commonly used in hospitals in emergency cases when a new pathogen appears – that is unknown until the present moment.

Thus we can also use chlorine in our and for our household. But it is very important what kind of chlorine we use. That is active chlorine or sodium hypochlorite.

What to look on when you buy disinfectant

Going on with our talk about chlorine, when you are buying a disinfectant (for surfaces), it is important that you are looking not only on the front label, but also on the back label – where it should say sodium hypochlorite (or, "active chlorine" on other products).

So, if you go to the supermarket and you buy a disinfectant on which's back label it says it contains sodium hypochlorite, then that product is good and can be used efficiently for disinfecting anything in your home – by using it according to the prospect.

How to make your own disinfectant

However, if you do not find such a disinfectant at the supermarket, then you can prepare your own at home and here is how.

You most certainly have a clothes' bleach product in your home. This is 100% made based on sodium hypochlorite

You should use about 0.65oz of that product to 33.8oz water. A small teaspoon for instance contains about 0.17oz of liquid.

As simple as this – and there you have your homemade house disinfectant.

Conclusion

Before entering a hospital guard or wash area, hands must be washed with soap and warm water for about twenty minutes. Handwashing eliminates around 99 percent of passing microorganisms. After that, if gloves are worn out or not, routine hygienic hand disinfection ought to take place to get rid of some succeeding transient flora and also to decrease the danger of the contamination originating out of properties that are resident.

The method of hands sanitization is of fantastic significance since the potency isn't only with all the alcohol.

In summary, hand sanitization is a significant process for employees to follow along with pharmaceutical and healthcare settings. Hand sanitization is just one of the chief procedures for preventing the spread of disease in pollution and hospitals inside pharmaceutical operations. This essential degree of control demands the usage of a successful hand sanitizer.

www.ingramcontent.com/pod-product-compliance
Lightning Source LLC
Chambersburg PA
CBHW070311220526
45465CB00004B/1845